Lifetime Medical Organizer

A Simple Guide to Organizing Matters of Life and Health How-To Instructions and Forms Included

Sandra J. Yorong with Richard Schuttler, Ph.D.

authorHOUSE®

AuthorHouse™
1663 Liberty Drive, Suite 200
Bloomington, IN 47403
www.authorhouse.com
Phone: 1-800-839-8640

First published by AuthorHouse 5/6/2008

ISBN: 978-1-4343-7684-8 (sc)

Library of Congress Control Number: 2008903831

Printed in the United States of America
Bloomington, Indiana

This book is printed on acid-free paper.

In loving memory of my Dad
Pedro Larot Yorong

Acknowledgments

This book was made possible by the encouragement of Richard Schuttler. Rich believed in my story and how it could help others. A journey is what you make of it, and I was blessed to be surrounded by encouraging friends and family that stood by me as I wrote the book. Bettelynn Cockett-Smith and Trish Chock filled the journey with enthusiasm and support. Anne Rautio, Kathy Mills, and Rhonda Thomas kept me laughing along the way. My church family lifted me up in prayer. Bart Koza found the time in his busy law practice to guide me in the legal areas. I am always grateful for the love and support of my mom, Betty Yorong, daughter Mandy Marumoto, and son-in-law Hayes Marumoto. Of course, the sunshine of my life, Haylie and Hunter, provided plenty of joy when I needed it most. Finally, I thank God for gracing me with His wisdom and for opening each new door of opportunity with every step of my journey.

Table of Contents

Chapter 1

My Story

Introduction

In January 2007, my father died of lung cancer at the age of 82. At the time of his diagnosis, his doctor told him he had between four and six months to live. Unfortunately, that was not the case. He passed away only three short months later. As one can imagine, my family struggled with a tidal wave of emotions during these months. While my father was not young, we did not expect him to pass away so soon. Several months before he was diagnosed, he appeared as healthy as he had ever been.

During that short period of three months, my family was confronted with many issues and concerns about how to manage my father's care and approaching death. We had not dealt with anything like this before, and there was much to manage with my father's appointments, medications, eating habits, legal affairs, medical bills, and other related matters. My siblings and I were challenged with managing the logistics and concerns of everyone involved, but most importantly we had to balance the respect we had for our parents and the decisions that only they could ultimately make. My story, and that of my family, is why and how I created the *Lifetime Medical Organizer*. This organizer provided our family with much peace of mind during a difficult time; it is my hope it will do the same for you.

My Father

My father, the second oldest of eight siblings, was the patriarch of his entire family, which included four children, four grandchildren, and two great grandchildren.

As a teenager, my father assumed responsibility for his younger siblings when his older brother entered the military. My father dropped out of high school to work and help his parents support the family. He made sure that his four younger brothers stayed out of trouble,

1

as well as protecting and providing for his two younger sisters. Both of his sisters adored him. One of my aunts once told me she was grateful to my father because he helped support her through college.

My father maintained that sense of responsibility until the end of his life. He was the one that everyone looked to for advice and guidance. He always made certain that his brothers provided for their families. If something happened to anyone in the family, one of the first telephone calls would be to my father. Until the end of his life, he remained close to his brothers and sisters and received the highest respect from his nieces and nephews. I remember at a family party, my male cousins were all sitting together having a good time when my father walked in—they all stood up to pay their respect and shook his hand. This is the kind of respect my father received from the family his whole life.

During my father's 82 years he made many friends. Even today, when I see them, they tell me my father "was a good man." Over the years, his friends have expressed how my father always had a kind word to share with them. My father did not do things in a grand way. He was a humble man, and his gestures of friendship were the same. As a father, he was strict, but he was also kind and gentle. He was more emotional than my mother; however, he had a way of balancing love and discipline that made us feel secure. He was our rock—not just to our family, but to the entire Yorong family. During his 82 years, many people turned to my father for love and guidance.

Even when he was in the hospital suffering, he still wanted to be strong for his family. It was understandable that everyone reached out to him and his family during his time of illness. My father was our family's hero!

My Mother

At the time of my father's death, my mother was 75 years old. She had been a homemaker married to my father for nearly 55 years. During these 55 years, she was a traditional Asian wife who managed the domestic duties and always took care of my father. My mother and father were inseparable, a true love story. It was understood that should my father take ill and need care during the marriage, she would be his primary caregiver.

My mother also came from a large family. She was the youngest of 10 children raised by traditional Chinese parents who preferred that she marry someone of the same race. Her father migrated from China to work in Hawaii; while there, he wed my grandmother as part of an arranged marriage. At the time they wed, my grandfather was 40 and my grandmother was 18. When my mother began dating my father, a man of Filipino descent, the relationship was not immediately accepted. It was only after my brother, the oldest sibling and only son in our family, was born that my Chinese grandparents began to accept my father. Over time, they embraced and respected my father for the good provider and husband he was.

My father often told us the story of how he had only 10 cents in his pocket the day he married my mother. Obviously, the relationship was meant to be, because my parents were soul mates and did everything together. For nearly 55 years, my father was the sole provider and my mother was a housewife. They ate breakfast together every morning, talked on the telephone almost every day during my father's lunch break at work, and always ate dinner together nightly. My mother did not drive, so they went everywhere together.

In their younger days, my parents would dance in the living room whenever a favorite song played on the television or radio. I would catch them snuggling on the sofa and even holding hands. After 55 years of marriage, we could still see the enormous love they had for each other. My mother tirelessly cared for my father during his illness. Even with all the pain and suffering my father went through in the hospital, he still managed to tell my mom she looked pretty.

As a small child growing up in Hawaii, my mother suffered an ear infection that was neglected. During that time, money was tight and my grandparents could not afford the necessary medical treatment. Due to the lack of medical care, the infection damaged my mother's eardrum and left her deaf in one ear. At the time of my father's illness, my mother's hearing capacity in her good ear declined to 15%. Although a hearing aid improved my mother's hearing slightly, it was still difficult for her to communicate with the health care providers who were giving my mother advice about my father. There were times when my mother, typically a strong and confident woman, became frustrated and emotionally distressed because of her hearing loss. She had a difficult time understanding the doctor's updates and recommendations. Since every decision about my father's care resided with my mother, communicating often became stressful as she tried to balance the emotions of watching her husband suffer with managing her own disability.

The Children

When my father was diagnosed with cancer, my older sister JoAnn and I lived near my parents. My older brother, Sanford, lived in Washington, and my youngest sister, Suzy, lived in California. When we received the news about our father, we were all busy with our own lives.

Like many families, our parents supported and provided help whenever we needed it. Often they spoiled us by putting our needs before their own. My parents did everything from baby-sitting to running errands, and most importantly they provided unconditional love that is far too immeasurable to describe. We could always count on them for anything without giving it a second thought.

My parents were typical grandparents and doted on their four grandchildren, often attending as many dance recitals and sporting events as they could. Ironically, the dynamics were similar in that my parents had three granddaughters (Mandy, Brandi, and Courtney) and one grandson (Taylor) in the same way they had three daughters and a son. There was never a month that left them without grandchildren visiting or sleeping over. One of my favorite memories of my father is taking out his ukulele and playing his favorite song to engage his grandchildren in song and dance. Great-grandchildren Haylie and Hunter became the absolute joy in my parents' lives. Despite the pain my father suffered during his last few months, he beamed with delight whenever his grandchildren and great-grandchildren visited.

During my father's illness, our family set aside our own needs and focused on what we needed to do as a family to adapt and support the changes that were fast approaching. Suddenly, daily hospital visits, eating on the run, chauffeuring a mother who does not drive, fielding countless telephone calls and e-mails, and attending to our own family matters became the new routine.

When a sudden or terminal illness confronts any family, *convenience* takes on a whole new meaning. Everyone involved needs to be working proactively and showing unselfish support. It can be easier said than done for some families, but our parents raised us to believe that family always comes first, and we kept the focus of working together to make things easier for them.

Quickly Cancer Takes Over

In April 2006, my mother told me that my father was suffering from the beginning stages of prostate cancer. Since the cancer was in the infancy stages, the doctors prescribed radiation treatments that began in July 2006. The doctors explained that the worst side effect my father would experience would be fatigue. My mother reassured us that this was not a serious threat.

Soon after the radiation treatments began, my father started complaining about pain in his back. With each passing month, the pain became more severe. When my mother asked the doctor to reexamine the pain my father was experiencing, the doctor discounted the pain as common geriatric progression and prescribed rehabilitation therapy. He also advised my father to accept this new stage of his life. Since my father was receiving radiation treatments during his therapy, we assumed that the treatments aggravated the pain, but did not think it was anything more serious.

After three months of witnessing my father's gradual weakening, inconsistent eating habits, more pain, and limited physical movement, my mother insisted that the doctors perform more tests. The doctors did perform another series of tests and said that the results would be available within a few weeks. That was just before the Thanksgiving holiday.

While waiting for the test results, another family tragedy occurred. We received heartbreaking news that my aunt, my mother's sister, who lived in California, had died. As my mother prepared to attend her sister's funeral in California, the doctor's office called to schedule an appointment to discuss the latest test results for my father. My parents decided to delay the appointment another week until after the Thanksgiving weekend and the funeral services for my aunt.

While my mother was out of town for my aunt's funeral, I cared for my father for three days during the Thanksgiving holiday. During that time, my father lost much of his appetite, and his physical movements became severely limited. In front of my father, I consistently expressed the brightest outlook and encouraged his every movement and eating habit. While my father slept, or during short drives to my home to replace personal belongings, I cried at witnessing the devastating decline of my father's health. I sensed that something was severely wrong. I became angry and questioned to myself why my father's doctor could not identify the source of the pain.

When my mother returned from California, during the ride home from the airport, I carefully explained the events that occurred over the Thanksgiving holiday. My siblings and I already discussed the possibility of changing doctors, and my mother agreed. As our family witnessed our father's decline, we felt frustrated and helpless. It was very difficult to believe that what was happening to my father was simply geriatric progression, as explained by his doctor. The following Tuesday we had our father admitted to the hospital under the care of a different doctor. The new doctor ordered tests, and the next day my father was released to await the results.

That evening after work, I stopped to visit my parents. That visit proved to be one of the hardest days of my life. My father was in the bathroom and I was sitting in the family room watching television when suddenly, my mom yelled, "Sandra, come quick. I need you!" My father hung over my mother like a limp tree branch as she struggled to hold him up. After 20 minutes of struggling to guide my father out of the bathroom with my mother, I personally called his new doctor. At that moment, the doctor confirmed that my father suffered from terminal lung cancer and had only a few months to live. The lung cancer was the reason for the pain in his back that had gone undiagnosed for several months.

I sobbed at the realization that my father would die soon—yet my father remained strong in spirit and tried to comfort me with his words. That night, we readmitted my father to the hospital, where he remained for several week before returning home under hospice care until his death. Ironically, my father's former doctor contacted us after discovering a mass from the x-rays, but it was too late—he had failed to detect it sooner, and we did not want anything to do with him.

Communicating to All

As my father's illness progressed, family and friends began to realize how serious the illness was. They became a constant source of love and support; however, with that came the difficult task of balancing my father's declining physical condition and everyone's emotions surrounding the situation. When a loved one's health declines, emotions can become highly charged, sometimes resulting in unintentional, hurtful, or resentful communication.

Where I live in Hawaii, extended families are a large part of the Hawaiian culture. This includes aunts, uncles, cousins, and friends. Trying to manage my father's health crisis and figuring out the best way of communicating updates to family and friends became a daunting task. Some wanted e-mail communication, others wanted telephone calls, and those who visited in the hospital wanted information from doctors repeated verbally on a daily basis. Communicating became a big concern. It was difficult handling my emotions as well as considering other people's feelings and staying focused on the important decisions that had to be made. Ultimately, every decision rested on my mother's approval.

During that period, my mother confronted many new challenges. For the many years she and my father were married, she always turned to him for help with making decisions. She was now forced to independently make major decisions for both of them. Because of her limited hearing, it was often difficult for my mother to understand the doctor's communications. This added to the stress in making the decisions she had to make. It was difficult for all of us; however, every decision fell upon my mother, and we were closely involved to help her.

Empathetic to my mother's hearing disability and trying to find a way to lessen the burden for her, I reassured her that she did not have to worry about the details of getting everything done. I began a plan to gather information. I wanted it to be in one place and in one concise manner. I wanted to be able to communicate to everyone in a consistent way with the most up-to-date information.

When communication is not managed effectively, lack of communication can lead to assumptions, stir all sorts of conflict, and create doubt, even though the communication is made with the best of intentions. This was the last thing we all wanted or needed during this difficult period, and I was determined to make it easier for all of us.

The Lifetime Medical Organizer Is Born

I needed a tool, a resource that could serve as a conduit to speak with logic and without emotion—or with as little as possible, considering the circumstances. I needed something that was easy to use and that many people could easily relate to about my father's care.

I searched through several retail bookstores and the Internet for an organizer that would be helpful. I expected that there would be many good ones to choose from—after all, people have to deal with these kinds of concerns every day. I found few organizers that would help in this situation, and those available seemed difficult to use. Many of the organizers that I examined appeared to want too much information; I found this intimidating, and it discouraged me from using them. Unless the user is analytical by nature, these types of organizers would mislead one to believe that data gathering is very complex and cumbersome.

So, I decided to create my own organizer that was simple to use, did not require huge amounts of data, and would provide the much-needed structure during our time of crisis. My mother came to rely on her organizer like a security blanket. It was the events leading up to my father's death and the encouragement I received from others that led me to create the Lifetime Medical Organizer.

Since my father's ordeal, I have received compliments and feedback from people about the ease of use and the simplicity that makes the Lifetime Medical Organizer so good. It is designed for simplicity and ease, as a starting point for others. People can customize their Lifetime Medical Organizers according to their own needs and take the steps to organizing their lives and health information *now* instead of waiting for a medical crisis to develop.

I am sharing my story so that you will be able to recognize what the Lifetime Medical Organizer can do for you as it relates to the love you have for your family and friends. In a time of crisis, it can help you identify what is important and create opportunities to keep it in focus. With my family, that importance was the love we had for our father. It is my hope that the Lifetime Medical Organizer will bring guidance and comfort to you and your family when it is needed the most.

Chapter 2

Lifetime Medical Organizer

The Lifetime Medical Organizer serves as a communication tool among family, friends, health care providers, and others. Think of it as a storage container that collectively holds your important information all in one place. Most people have what I call a "chop suey" approach to managing important information. For example, you may have legal documents safely tucked away in a safe-deposit box at the bank. Your medicine may be in your medicine cabinet or somewhere near a sink on a countertop. If you recorded your medicine intake, you probably have it posted on the refrigerator or family bulletin board. Other types of financial, insurance, and personal data remain in a folder in a file cabinet or stored in a computer. Your doctors' business cards are lying somewhere on a desk. Does this sound like you?

During a critical or emergency situation, imagine the problems you create for your loved ones when they have to find all of this information. By having the information assembled in your Lifetime Medical Organizer, you lessen such problems in what is going to be a stressful and emotional time for everyone involved.

The Communication Tool

Your Lifetime Medical Organizer is a simple tool. How you use it determines how effective it will be to communicate to your loved ones. I like to summarize poor communication with the phrase "lack of communication leads to assumptions." When there is limited information for someone to decide the proper outcome or interpret the correct meaning, assumptions can sometimes suggest the wrong intent. In the same way, not providing enough information to aid in your care may create conflicts or doubt among family members when they have to make decisions on your behalf.

When your medical information is not properly organized, there is the potential for delayed medical attention until you, or someone in your family, provides the necessary information. Like many things in life, we take for granted that someone will have this information readily available when we need it most. By putting together your Lifetime Medical Organizer, you minimize the risk that comes with being unprepared. You also make it easier for loved ones in time of need. It makes better sense to be prepared today by developing your information and placing it in your Lifetime Medical Organizer.

Getting Started

Begin thinking about how to build your Lifetime Medical Organizer. The most important thing for you to keep in mind is what you should communicate and what others will need to know when you are not able to respond. How well do you want to communicate your information to others and what will they need during an emergency or critical situation? The information you provide should be user friendly for quick access to your information.

If you will be using your Lifetime Medical Organizer to manage daily and monthly information, your information should always remain current. However, if you are using the Lifetime Medical Organizer as a reference binder for only emergencies, make sure to review and update your information at least once a year or immediately after any change is made to your situation. Remember, the Lifetime Medical Organizer is only as useful as the information you record in it. If you have outdated information such as medicine that you are no longer taking, how useful would that information be to your doctors during a current emergency?

I have provided you with the forms I believe are essential for you to create your own Lifetime Medical Organizer. Each form comes with a description of importance, simple how-to steps to get you started, and questions to consider. As you complete each form, you will begin to develop a better understanding of how to use it. Once the forms are completed and you insert the right documents, you can further customize your organizer with other relevant information you believe will be needed by others to help you.

There is no such thing as too much information if it is organized. And there is no right or wrong way of building your Lifetime Medical Organizer. It is always better to have more relevant information than not enough. I have provided what I believe is essential, but you are the best person to decide how much information belongs in your organizer.

When following the steps to building your information, imagine you are unconscious at the time of an emergency. Your Lifetime Medical Organizer becomes your voice and must speak to everyone who will need to know information on your behalf. You will want to feel confident and have peace of mind in knowing that your Lifetime Medical Organizer will turn into your best friend when you need to rely on it the most.

On completion of your information, share it with the important people in your life. Explain the importance of the contents and share your intentions in case you are not able to communicate with them later. The conversation will leave you with greater peace of mind, knowing that you are well prepared for an emergency or crisis and that the information in your Lifetime Medical Organizer will provide needed guidance for those who may have to make serious decisions on your behalf.

My Hope for You

I created the Lifetime Medical Organizer for my parents during a critical and difficult time. My siblings and I wanted my mother to avoid the burden of managing my father's affairs so that she could focus on tending to his needs during his last few months. We could see the commitment and love my mother had for my father while he slowly weakened, and that was what mattered most to her at the time.

We wanted to honor the depth of love our parents built with 55 years of marriage, and the best way to do that was to allow them to love each other without distraction. Of course, this goal transferred the burden of paperwork, planning, and communication to my sister and me, even while we were still managing our own personal obligations. In addition, we were responsible for conveying updates to all family and friends concerned with my father's health. Luckily, the organizer helped us to manage these tasks easier than we could have otherwise.

It is stressful to gather essential data during a difficult period in the hospital. Our family shared the duties of spending every day and night with my mother at the hospital, meeting with doctors, talking with relatives who were near and far, sending e-mail updates, caring for my mother's well-being, and managing the administration of my father's last wishes all at once. The organizer kept everyone's focus and communication consistent during this difficult period and provided much-needed peace of mind. It is my hope that your Lifetime Medical Organizer will bring your family the same benefits as it did to ours.

Chapter 3

Real Stories

Before you begin developing your Lifetime Medical Organizer, I want to share several stories from my family and friends that can help highlight the importance of creating one. They say that your best critics are your family and friends because they keep you grounded and provide blunt honesty. Fortunately, I do not have a shortage of family and friends who provided me with that honesty. Their input became very valuable as I began developing this organizer.

I am fortunate that I did not have a truly harsh critic in the bunch, but I appreciated the honest feedback they provided. My friends allowed me the opportunity to share each of their "best practice" approaches for using their own Lifetime Medical Organizer.

Can We All Get Along?

In the early stages of developing the Lifetime Medical Organizer for my family, I also created an organizer for my best friend, Bettelynn, whose mother was ill. Bettelynn had lost her father the year before, and her mother's health was declining. Because of dementia and geriatric progression, her mother could no longer care for herself. Bettelynn comes from a family of eight siblings who are scattered across the country. Each one had a different opinion on the best way for managing the care for their mother. Eventually, Bettelynn's youngest sister, Cecily, volunteered to become the primary caregiver, and their mother moved into her home. Cecily assumed the task of communicating updates and managing medical and personal information for her family while balancing the time needed to physically care for her mother.

Equipped with their Lifetime Medical Organizer, Cecily gained peace of mind knowing that the information was easily available. She took the organizer to doctor visits and kept it close when family visited. When Cecily gave the Lifetime Medical Organizer to the hospital staff, they expressed appreciation for the comprehensive approach to managing her mother's care. The staff delighted in the easy access to information needed to make copies of legal documents, contacts, medicine information, and journal notes that provided a wealth of information for staff and doctors changing with shift duties.

The Lifetime Medical Organizer reduced the number of questions and provided reassurance to other siblings. All of the necessary information was easily available for review. Some scanned and sent documents by e-mail to family out-of-state so they could be included in the conversations and decision making. In this way, their Lifetime Medical Organizer centered the family's focus on their mother's care rather than time spent on distractions involving details of care management in the emergency room.

Help! Call 9-1-1

Anne, a registered nurse at a local hospital, experienced many situations in which adult children and family members accompanied a loved one to the emergency room for immediate care. Sometimes there was a delay in providing care because the medical staff was trying to get information about the patient. Anne explained that adult children and family members seldom have the necessary information available at a moment's notice during an emergency. Usually, there is standard information like health and medical coverage and the name of the family doctor, but other important data may not be readily available for the attending doctor.

The Lifetime Medical Organizer serves as an immediate resource to notify emergency health care providers about recent medical conditions and medications. Legal documents become even more important if the situation becomes life-or-death. Important contact names and numbers are available for immediate notification. It should not be taken for granted that the person with all the contact, medical, and legal information will be the same person accompanying the patient in need of emergency care. Many times emergencies occur in the middle of the night or during the weekend, and having the correct information can become critically important.

Long-Distance Assistance

Richard and Barbara are siblings and the only surviving members of their immediate family. Both of their parents died of heart attacks—father at age 60 and mother at age 76. Richard considers the form for recording family medical history to be an important reference for future doctor visits. In addition, Richard and Barbara live in different states, and Richard's career requires much travel throughout the United States and to other countries. Neither is married or have children. The Lifetime Medical Organizer has prompted an increased awareness that they each should have their life and health information available for the other's benefit should the need arise.

The Lifetime Medical Organizer increased the urgency for each to prepare legal documents, especially a durable power of attorney and health care directive, to which neither had given a second thought because of their single status. Since Richard travels often, the Lifetime Medical Organizer serves as a conduit between him and his sister in case of an emergency. Both also keep their closest friends informed about their own Lifetime Medical Organizer and where it can be found.

Sibling Support

Stan and his siblings share in managing their elderly mother's life and health information. One manages his mother's day-to-day care and medications. Another oversees the legal documents, while another is confidant to his mother's financial situation. Finally, the youngest, who is the appointed executor of his mother's estate, lives near her in Philadelphia. Stan lives in Hawaii and provides long-distance input. Although Stan and his siblings share in caring for their mother, it is more of an individual approach rather than a collective effort.

The approach of sharing the responsibilities can occasionally cause frustrations. This approach needs constant collaboration from everyone for every situation. When Stan's mother was admitted to the hospital for a short time, managing her affairs appeared like a maze of doors that opened and shut, with each sibling handling different needs. Since Stan's mother does not need constant care or attention, Stan wants to immediately incorporate the Lifetime Medical Organizer in his mother's life and health matters. In the future, they can better manage their mother's affairs, and each will know where to find the needed information. This collective organization will minimize a communication breakdown and provide better care for their mother.

Helping Others

I work in the financial planning and investment industry, where my work includes managing and organizing clients' financial affairs. As I establish long-term relationships with my clients, I gain a better understanding of the changing needs that come with life-cycle changes—from having children, changing careers, retiring, and other life events. The Lifetime Medical Organizer serves as a value-added component to financial or estate planning with a direct link to assets and investments. This is especially true during a time of medical or personal crisis. Legal documents may be required for medical decision making, and excessive medical bills may need the liquidation of certain financial assets. For these and other reasons the Lifetime Medical Organizer should be an essential part of everyone's planning. Establishing the organizer and discussing it with your financial advisor strengthens the value-added service between the client and advisor.

Real Stories

The examples above are each different, yet the Lifetime Medical Organizer accommodates many situations. As your own story develops, how do you want it to be played out? Putting together your own Lifetime Medical Organizer now will make that story better than it would be otherwise. The best gifts in life are those that help others. The Lifetime Medical Organizer will help you and your loved ones for years to come.

Chapter 4

Emergency Telephone Directory Form

Imagine having to search your parents' home, while they are hospitalized, to find important telephone numbers for people they want you to call. Would you be able to quickly find your parents' cell phone or have access to their computer? Sometimes a computer needs a password that you may not know, and most cell phone numbers do not easily show any special priority for emergencies. These are just some of the delays that may conflict with your attempts to find the information you need. By having a printed emergency telephone directory in your easy-to-find Lifetime Medical Organizer, you have available the contact information for everyone who needs it quickly and easily.

My Experience

When my father was ill and dying of cancer, our emergency telephone directory came in handy. This was particularly important in our case because my mother did not know how to use a cell phone. During the years when pagers were popular, I remember a funny story about my mother trying to page my daughter Mandy. After several attempts without a return call from Mandy, my mother called me slightly annoyed. She explained that she had called Mandy's pager number and followed the voice instructions. Later, we found out that my mother had spoken the numbers instead of pressing the keypad on the telephone.

When elderly people are involved, do not assume that they are familiar with how to use the latest technology, such as computers and cell phones. Help others so they can help you. A printed copy in the Lifetime Medical Organizer is always a handy reference.

How To

List the names, addresses, and contact information for those in your life that you want contacted immediately if a crisis occurs. You may want to consider listing them in the priority you want them contacted. For example, if you have four children and prefer to have your youngest child contacted first, do not list your children in the order of birth. Or, you may decide that you want your best friend or significant other notified before your children or other family members. You may also prefer to contact a co-worker before certain friends and extended family members.

Show a priority next to each contact so the person reading your directory can easily understand your preference. Instinctively, most people will begin calling the first person listed on the top of the form. If you are going to be away from your job for a period of time, it would be helpful to list the contact person at your job to be notified of your absence. Your employer may need certain paperwork to be completed to ensure that medical, insurance, or disability benefits continue during your absence.

Questions to Consider

• Who do I want contacted during an emergency?
• What priority do I want my contacts called?

EMERGENCY TELEPHONE DIRECTORY

NAME & ADDRESS	RELATIONSHIP	CONTACT INFORMATION
Name	Address	Home
	City/State/Zip	Work
Relationship	Email	Cell
Name	Address	Home
	City/State/Zip	Work
Relationship	Email	Cell
Name	Address	Home
	City/State/Zip	Work
Relationship	Email	Cell
Name	Address	Home
	City/State/Zip	Work
Relationship	Email	Cell
Name	Address	Home
	City/State/Zip	Work
Relationship	Email	Cell
Name	Address	Home
	City/State/Zip	Work
Relationship	Email	Cell
Name	Address	Home
	City/State/Zip	Work
Relationship	Email	Cell

EMERGENCY TELEPHONE DIRECTORY

NAME & ADDRESS	RELATIONSHIP	CONTACT INFORMATION
Name Relationship	Address City/State/Zip Email	Home Work Cell
Name Relationship	Address City/State/Zip Email	Home Work Cell
Name Relationship	Address City/State/Zip Email	Home Work Cell
Name Relationship	Address City/State/Zip Email	Home Work Cell
Name Relationship	Address City/State/Zip Email	Home Work Cell
Name Relationship	Address City/State/Zip Email	Home Work Cell
Name Relationship	Address City/State/Zip Email	Home Work Cell

EMERGENCY TELEPHONE DIRECTORY

NAME & ADDRESS	RELATIONSHIP	CONTACT INFORMATION
Name	Address	Home
	City/State/Zip	Work
Relationship	Email	Cell
Name	Address	Home
	City/State/Zip	Work
Relationship	Email	Cell
Name	Address	Home
	City/State/Zip	Work
Relationship	Email	Cell
Name	Address	Home
	City/State/Zip	Work
Relationship	Email	Cell
Name	Address	Home
	City/State/Zip	Work
Relationship	Email	Cell
Name	Address	Home
	City/State/Zip	Work
Relationship	Email	Cell
Name	Address	Home
	City/State/Zip	Work
Relationship	Email	Cell

EMERGENCY TELEPHONE DIRECTORY

NAME & ADDRESS	RELATIONSHIP	CONTACT INFORMATION
Name Relationship	Address City/State/Zip Email	Home Work Cell
Name Relationship	Address City/State/Zip Email	Home Work Cell
Name Relationship	Address City/State/Zip Email	Home Work Cell
Name Relationship	Address City/State/Zip Email	Home Work Cell
Name Relationship	Address City/State/Zip Email	Home Work Cell
Name Relationship	Address City/State/Zip Email	Home Work Cell
Name Relationship	Address City/State/Zip Email	Home Work Cell

Chapter 5

Doctor Directory Form

Your Lifetime Medical Organizer provides you with a form to show your doctors separately from those in your Emergency Telephone Directory form. At a quick glance, it is easier for the user to find the information associated with your doctors and how to contact them in one dedicated place. Hospital staff and emergency personnel may want to contact your family doctor immediately, and this section guides them with ease. In addition, the directory will provide a quick summary of the types of doctors that provide treatment to you.

My Experience

My father had several doctors treating him at the same time. There was his family doctor, the attending doctor at the hospital, the cardiologist, and the radiologist. It became increasingly difficult to associate daily and weekly updates with each doctor when things happened so quickly. It was also difficult for friends and family to follow the progress reports when they could not easily identify the doctor's specialty.

By listing the doctors and their specialties in one convenient location in the Lifetime Medical Organizer, it is easier to glance back and forth when reading appointment and meeting notes. After a while, my family had an easier time following updates because of this form.

How To

List the names, addresses, telephone numbers, and specialties for every doctor. It is also important to show the after-hours telephone numbers in case you need to call during non-business hours. If you work closely with an assistant or junior medical assistant within your doctor's practice, make sure to list this person's name on your Doctor Directory form as well.

Another good idea is to attach your doctors' business cards to this section.

Questions to Consider

- How many doctors do I have?
- Are there other health care providers I should include in this directory?

DOCTOR DIRECTORY

DOCTOR'S NAME & ADDRESS	SPECIALTY	CONTACT INFO
Name Address City/State/Zip		Office Fax Cell After Hours Email Other
Name Address City/State/Zip		Office Fax Cell After Hours Email Other
Name Address City/State/Zip		Office Fax Cell After Hours Email Other
Name Address City/State/Zip		Office Fax Cell After Hours Email Other
Name Address City/State/Zip		Office Fax Cell After Hours Email Other
Name Address City/State/Zip		Office Fax Cell After Hours Email Other

DOCTOR DIRECTORY

DOCTOR'S NAME & ADDRESS	SPECIALTY	CONTACT INFO
Name Address City/State/Zip		Office Fax Cell After Hours Email Other
Name Address City/State/Zip		Office Fax Cell After Hours Email Other
Name Address City/State/Zip		Office Fax Cell After Hours Email Other
Name Address City/State/Zip		Office Fax Cell After Hours Email Other
Name Address City/State/Zip		Office Fax Cell After Hours Email Other
Name Address City/State/Zip		Office Fax Cell After Hours Email Other

DOCTOR DIRECTORY

DOCTOR'S NAME & ADDRESS	SPECIALTY	CONTACT INFO	
Name		Office	
		Fax	
Address		Cell	
		After Hours	
		Email	
City/State/Zip		Other	
Name		Office	
		Fax	
Address		Cell	
		After Hours	
		Email	
City/State/Zip		Other	
Name		Office	
		Fax	
Address		Cell	
		After Hours	
		Email	
City/State/Zip		Other	
Name		Office	
		Fax	
Address		Cell	
		After Hours	
		Email	
City/State/Zip		Other	
Name		Office	
		Fax	
Address		Cell	
		After Hours	
		Email	
City/State/Zip		Other	
Name		Office	
		Fax	
Address		Cell	
		After Hours	
		Email	
City/State/Zip		Other	

DOCTOR DIRECTORY

DOCTOR'S NAME & ADDRESS	SPECIALTY	CONTACT INFO
Name Address City/State/Zip		Office Fax Cell After Hours Email Other
Name Address City/State/Zip		Office Fax Cell After Hours Email Other
Name Address City/State/Zip		Office Fax Cell After Hours Email Other
Name Address City/State/Zip		Office Fax Cell After Hours Email Other
Name Address City/State/Zip		Office Fax Cell After Hours Email Other
Name Address City/State/Zip		Office Fax Cell After Hours Email Other

Chapter 6

Other Important Contacts Form

Family, friends, and doctors are not the only people for whom you should include contact information in your Lifetime Medical Organizer. Your life is filled with many obligations that will continue regardless of your condition. Bills need to be paid, household chores need attention, checks have to be deposited, and professional associates locally or long-distance may need to be identified or contacted. If you are unable to take care of your own needs for any period of time, the person you have identified to help you will step into the role of managing your affairs. Listing other contacts will provide assistance to this person in knowing where you would want her or him to start.

My Experience

Since my mother was in good health during my father's illness, we did not worry about the necessary contacts or essential matters that needed updating. However, should anything happen to my mother, I am appointed her power of attorney and would know where to begin only because I will use this form from her organizer. In situations where you do not know who to contact, it becomes time-consuming to review or discover every utility bill, bank statement, or file box for assembling the pieces of the puzzle.

My father retired many years ago, and although my mother knew the name of the company he retired from, she did not have current contact information. Over time, the company and its employees changed with new ownership. Changes of this sort can delay the process for updating pension and benefits information. When you are dealing with time differences, your own work schedule, and sorting through documents, delays may occur. Unfortunately, these delays can sometimes cause interruptions with continuous income streams from pension distributions, social security checks, and other types of income sources for the surviving spouse or loved ones.

How To

For each section on the form in the organizer, specifically list the company, branch office, contact person, telephone, and e-mail contacts. Consider the Account Type section as a user guide only. To avoid identity theft, if you plan on storing your Lifetime Medical Organizer somewhere easily accessible to all, DO NOT include confidential account information like account numbers, user names, passwords, etc.

By checking the box associated with the account type, you are only pointing out where you do business and what types of accounts you have with a professional. The person helping you will contact the appropriate business or professional shown on your form for further help. You may also want to attach the company's business card in this section. The more information and people you include in this section, the easier it will make it for the person helping with your affairs.

Questions to Consider

• Who should be contacted in case of an emergency, hospitalization, or death?

• Would my workplace or the company I retired from need to be contacted to ensure continuity of medical or death benefits?

OTHER IMPORTANT CONTACTS

NAME & ADDRESS	CONTACT NUMBERS	ACCOUNT TYPE	
Name	Office	☐	Bank Accounts
		☐	Investments
Title	Fax	☐	Auto Insurance
		☐	Homeowners Insurance
Company	Cell	☐	Life Insurance
		☐	Legal (Wills, Trusts, etc.)
Email	Other	☐	Other

NAME & ADDRESS	CONTACT NUMBERS	ACCOUNT TYPE	
Name	Office	☐	Bank Accounts
		☐	Investments
Title	Fax	☐	Auto Insurance
		☐	Homeowners Insurance
Company	Cell	☐	Life Insurance
		☐	Legal (Wills, Trusts, etc.)
Email	Other	☐	Other

NAME & ADDRESS	CONTACT NUMBERS	ACCOUNT TYPE	
Name	Office	☐	Bank Accounts
		☐	Investments
Title	Fax	☐	Auto Insurance
		☐	Homeowners Insurance
Company	Cell	☐	Life Insurance
		☐	Legal (Wills, Trusts, etc.)
Email	Other	☐	Other

NAME & ADDRESS	CONTACT NUMBERS	ACCOUNT TYPE	
Name	Office	☐	Bank Accounts
		☐	Investments
Title	Fax	☐	Auto Insurance
		☐	Homeowners Insurance
Company	Cell	☐	Life Insurance
		☐	Legal (Wills, Trusts, etc.)
Email	Other	☐	Other

NAME & ADDRESS	CONTACT NUMBERS	ACCOUNT TYPE	
Name	Office	☐	Bank Accounts
		☐	Investments
Title	Fax	☐	Auto Insurance
		☐	Homeowners Insurance
Company	Cell	☐	Life Insurance
		☐	Legal (Wills, Trusts, etc.)
Email	Other	☐	Other

OTHER IMPORTANT CONTACTS

NAME & ADDRESS	CONTACT NUMBERS	ACCOUNT TYPE
Name	Office	Bank Accounts
		Investments
Title	Fax	Auto Insurance
		Homeowners Insurance
Company	Cell	Life Insurance
		Legal (Wills, Trusts, etc.)
Email	Other	Other

NAME & ADDRESS	CONTACT NUMBERS	ACCOUNT TYPE
Name	Office	Bank Accounts
		Investments
Title	Fax	Auto Insurance
		Homeowners Insurance
Company	Cell	Life Insurance
		Legal (Wills, Trusts, etc.)
Email	Other	Other

NAME & ADDRESS	CONTACT NUMBERS	ACCOUNT TYPE
Name	Office	Bank Accounts
		Investments
Title	Fax	Auto Insurance
		Homeowners Insurance
Company	Cell	Life Insurance
		Legal (Wills, Trusts, etc.)
Email	Other	Other

NAME & ADDRESS	CONTACT NUMBERS	ACCOUNT TYPE
Name	Office	Bank Accounts
		Investments
Title	Fax	Auto Insurance
		Homeowners Insurance
Company	Cell	Life Insurance
		Legal (Wills, Trusts, etc.)
Email	Other	Other

NAME & ADDRESS	CONTACT NUMBERS	ACCOUNT TYPE
Name	Office	Bank Accounts
		Investments
Title	Fax	Auto Insurance
		Homeowners Insurance
Company	Cell	Life Insurance
		Legal (Wills, Trusts, etc.)
Email	Other	Other

OTHER IMPORTANT CONTACTS

NAME & ADDRESS	CONTACT NUMBERS	ACCOUNT TYPE
Name	Office	☐ Bank Accounts
		☐ Investments
Title	Fax	☐ Auto Insurance
		☐ Homeowners Insurance
Company	Cell	☐ Life Insurance
		☐ Legal (Wills, Trusts, etc.)
Email	Other	☐ Other

NAME & ADDRESS	CONTACT NUMBERS	ACCOUNT TYPE
Name	Office	☐ Bank Accounts
		☐ Investments
Title	Fax	☐ Auto Insurance
		☐ Homeowners Insurance
Company	Cell	☐ Life Insurance
		☐ Legal (Wills, Trusts, etc.)
Email	Other	☐ Other

NAME & ADDRESS	CONTACT NUMBERS	ACCOUNT TYPE
Name	Office	☐ Bank Accounts
		☐ Investments
Title	Fax	☐ Auto Insurance
		☐ Homeowners Insurance
Company	Cell	☐ Life Insurance
		☐ Legal (Wills, Trusts, etc.)
Email	Other	☐ Other

NAME & ADDRESS	CONTACT NUMBERS	ACCOUNT TYPE
Name	Office	☐ Bank Accounts
		☐ Investments
Title	Fax	☐ Auto Insurance
		☐ Homeowners Insurance
Company	Cell	☐ Life Insurance
		☐ Legal (Wills, Trusts, etc.)
Email	Other	☐ Other

NAME & ADDRESS	CONTACT NUMBERS	ACCOUNT TYPE
Name	Office	☐ Bank Accounts
		☐ Investments
Title	Fax	☐ Auto Insurance
		☐ Homeowners Insurance
Company	Cell	☐ Life Insurance
		☐ Legal (Wills, Trusts, etc.)
Email	Other	☐ Other

OTHER IMPORTANT CONTACTS

NAME & ADDRESS	CONTACT NUMBERS	ACCOUNT TYPE
Name	Office	☐ Bank Accounts
		☐ Investments
Title	Fax	☐ Auto Insurance
		☐ Homeowners Insurance
Company	Cell	☐ Life Insurance
		☐ Legal (Wills, Trusts, etc.)
Email	Other	☐ Other

NAME & ADDRESS	CONTACT NUMBERS	ACCOUNT TYPE
Name	Office	☐ Bank Accounts
		☐ Investments
Title	Fax	☐ Auto Insurance
		☐ Homeowners Insurance
Company	Cell	☐ Life Insurance
		☐ Legal (Wills, Trusts, etc.)
Email	Other	☐ Other

NAME & ADDRESS	CONTACT NUMBERS	ACCOUNT TYPE
Name	Office	☐ Bank Accounts
		☐ Investments
Title	Fax	☐ Auto Insurance
		☐ Homeowners Insurance
Company	Cell	☐ Life Insurance
		☐ Legal (Wills, Trusts, etc.)
Email	Other	☐ Other

NAME & ADDRESS	CONTACT NUMBERS	ACCOUNT TYPE
Name	Office	☐ Bank Accounts
		☐ Investments
Title	Fax	☐ Auto Insurance
		☐ Homeowners Insurance
Company	Cell	☐ Life Insurance
		☐ Legal (Wills, Trusts, etc.)
Email	Other	☐ Other

NAME & ADDRESS	CONTACT NUMBERS	ACCOUNT TYPE
Name	Office	☐ Bank Accounts
		☐ Investments
Title	Fax	☐ Auto Insurance
		☐ Homeowners Insurance
Company	Cell	☐ Life Insurance
		☐ Legal (Wills, Trusts, etc.)
Email	Other	☐ Other

Chapter 7

Medicine Prescription Record Form

Prescription records are an essential part of the Lifetime Medical Organizer. It tells the reader the medication prescribed by your doctor. If you have different medication prescribed by different doctors, consider sharing your prescription record with each doctor, to be incorporated in their files. You can take it one step further by providing your doctor with a copy of your Medicine Prescription Record form to reference during future office visits.

Often doctors prescribe medicine for specific treatments without knowing that you may be taking other prescribed medication for treatment from other doctors. Unfortunately, some medicines do have adverse reactions to others. Do not assume that your doctor is aware of all the medicine you are taking, even though you may have mentioned it in the past. Keep in mind that the information you may have provided your doctor previously may now be outdated.

My Experience

Pharmacists are trained to analyze reactions, or counter-reactions, from prescribed medicine. My father had up to five prescriptions at one time. I asked our local pharmacist, who filled my father's prescriptions, to conduct an analysis of all the medicines to discover any risk for side effects. We gained a greater level of comfort to learn that my father's medicines did not conflict with one another. This also gave us greater confidence in the health care that was provided to him. The pharmacist further educated me by providing more detail for each medicine. During this brief meeting, the pharmacist allowed me to ask questions and express my concerns as well.

My friend Dave shared with me that during his father's illness, he helped manage both of his parents' medical affairs. Dave counted 25 prescriptions between his parents. It was difficult for him to remember them all until he began listing them in an organized manner. When Dave shared the list with the doctors, they were amazed at the amount of medicine both parents consumed. The list helped the doctors become more aware of all current prescriptions that in turn provided better health care for both parents.

How To

List the names of every medicine, dosage, frequency, and purpose for taking each on your form. In addition, list any allergies and include the computer printout statements that your pharmacist provides when filling prescriptions. The statement explains the purpose for the medicine, possible side effects, and other information important for you to know. Should you or your loved one suffer an adverse reaction from the medicine, you can quickly refer back to the prescription statement for information about the symptoms or side effects. Remember to always consult your doctor immediately if you or your loved one detects any changes resulting from medicine that may pose a health risk.

IMPORTANT

It is important to keep this section up-to-date because prescriptions change. This section can quickly become obsolete and perhaps useless if it does not show the most current prescriptions when you need to rely on it most. Literally, the information in this section can help save your life!

Questions to Consider

- Should I take all of my medicines to my pharmacist and have them analyzed together?
- Have I shared my medicine information with all of my doctors?

MEDICINE PRESCRIPTION RECORD

List any allergies to medications.

NAME OF MEDICINE	PRESCRIPTION	PURPOSE
Brand	Dosage	
Prescribed by	Frequency	
Brand	Dosage	
Prescribed by	Frequency	
Brand	Dosage	
Prescribed by	Frequency	
Brand	Dosage	
Prescribed by	Frequency	
Brand	Dosage	
Prescribed by	Frequency	
Brand	Dosage	
Prescribed by	Frequency	
Brand	Dosage	
Prescribed by	Frequency	
Brand	Dosage	
Prescribed by	Frequency	
Brand	Dosage	
Prescribed by	Frequency	

MEDICINE PRESCRIPTION RECORD

List any allergies to medications.

_____
_____
_____
_____

NAME OF MEDICINE	PRESCRIPTION	PURPOSE
Brand Prescribed by	Dosage Frequency	
Brand Prescribed by	Dosage Frequency	
Brand Prescribed by	Dosage Frequency	
Brand Prescribed by	Dosage Frequency	
Brand Prescribed by	Dosage Frequency	
Brand Prescribed by	Dosage Frequency	
Brand Prescribed by	Dosage Frequency	
Brand Prescribed by	Dosage Frequency	
Brand Prescribed by	Dosage Frequency	

MEDICINE PRESCRIPTION RECORD

List any allergies to medications.

_____

_____

_____

_____

NAME OF MEDICINE	PRESCRIPTION	PURPOSE
Brand	Dosage	
Prescribed by	Frequency	
Brand	Dosage	
Prescribed by	Frequency	
Brand	Dosage	
Prescribed by	Frequency	
Brand	Dosage	
Prescribed by	Frequency	
Brand	Dosage	
Prescribed by	Frequency	
Brand	Dosage	
Prescribed by	Frequency	
Brand	Dosage	
Prescribed by	Frequency	
Brand	Dosage	
Prescribed by	Frequency	
Brand	Dosage	
Prescribed by	Frequency	

MEDICINE PRESCRIPTION RECORD

List any allergies to medications.

_____
_____
_____
_____

NAME OF MEDICINE	PRESCRIPTION	PURPOSE
Brand Prescribed by	Dosage Frequency	
Brand Prescribed by	Dosage Frequency	
Brand Prescribed by	Dosage Frequency	
Brand Prescribed by	Dosage Frequency	
Brand Prescribed by	Dosage Frequency	
Brand Prescribed by	Dosage Frequency	
Brand Prescribed by	Dosage Frequency	
Brand Prescribed by	Dosage Frequency	
Brand Prescribed by	Dosage Frequency	

Chapter 8

Daily Medicine Consumption Form

Chapter 7 helped you organize your medicine prescriptions. Now it is time to document your daily medicine consumption. Some medicine is prescribed to be taken with meals, while others are to be taken on an empty stomach. The purpose of this form is to note the time of day you consumed your medicine and keep you on schedule to avoid confusion. In a world where multitasking allows one to manage several tasks at once, applying some association may work for a single medicine. However, imagine having to consume four or five different pills, capsules, or fluids daily, each at different times of the day and incorporating some routine from memory. It would be difficult for a *healthy* person to remember, let alone someone not feeling well or partially incapacitated.

My Experience

My father consumed up to five different medicines each day. During his hospital stay, the nurses oversaw and recorded his medicine intake. When my father came home, my mother became his caretaker and assumed the responsibility of watching and managing his medicine. I quickly realized the challenges my mother confronted. After all, it was an emotionally difficult time for her. Although she and my father appreciated visitors, she had interruptions with frequent telephone calls and visits from family and friends during the week, which caused minor distractions.

Initially, to manage my father's medicine consumption, my mother wrote reminders on little yellow sticky notes and other pieces of paper, but this practice made me uncomfortable. I recognized that her approach could confuse her just as much as it was confusing me. As soon as I created the Daily Medicine Consumption form and shared it with my mother, she felt more in control of managing my father's medicine.

When confronted with a major illness or injury, small concerns can potentially develop into bigger problems over time. If left unmanaged or unorganized, these problems could require extra effort that takes away from spending time with your loved one. My mother was relieved to know that this area of my father's care was well organized.

How To

List all prescribed medicine you consume on a daily basis and show both the dosage and frequency for each. Next, record each time of day you take the medicine. Remember, this form is only as useful as the information you provide. It is important for you to develop some routine to make recordkeeping habit-forming. You may want to consider keeping this form separate from your Lifetime Medical Organizer and near the medicine cabinet, sink, or wherever you keep your medicine. However, remember to keep the form where it is easy for others to locate. If you choose this approach, insert the completed form into the binder at the end of each week before starting a new one.

This form is not intended to hold you to a rigid schedule. Rather, it is simply a method to help make recordkeeping for dispensed medicine easier. This form can also be helpful to others if you should happen to experience a problem that results in an adverse reaction from certain medicine consumption.

Paramedics and hospital emergency care providers may be able to respond more quickly to your needs if they know what you were doing when the situation occurred and what medicine you recently consumed. In an emergency situation, the sooner medical care providers can accurately assess what has happened, the faster they can help you.

Questions to Consider

- What area of my home is the easiest place to assemble my medicine and Daily Medicine Consumption form?
- Could someone quickly and easily identify what prescriptions I have and when I take my daily medicine?

DAILY MEDICINE CONSUMPTION

Medicine	Date	Sunday	Monday	Tuesday	Wednesday	Thursday	Friday	Saturday
Brand/Dosage		am am	am am	am am	am am	am am	am am	am am
How often?		pm pm	pm pm	pm pm	pm pm	pm pm	pm pm	pm pm
Brand/Dosage		am am	am am	am am	am am	am am	am am	am am
How often?		pm pm	pm pm	pm pm	pm pm	pm pm	pm pm	pm pm
Brand/Dosage		am am	am am	am am	am am	am am	am am	am am
How often?		pm pm	pm pm	pm pm	pm pm	pm pm	pm pm	pm pm
Brand/Dosage		am am	am am	am am	am am	am am	am am	am am
How often?		pm pm	pm pm	pm pm	pm pm	pm pm	pm pm	pm pm
Brand/Dosage		am am	am am	am am	am am	am am	am am	am am
How often?		pm pm	pm pm	pm pm	pm pm	pm pm	pm pm	pm pm

DAILY MEDICINE CONSUMPTION

Medicine / Date	Sunday	Monday	Tuesday	Wednesday	Thursday	Friday	Saturday
Brand/Dosage							
How often?	am pm	am pm	am pm	am pm	am pm	am pm	am pm
Brand/Dosage							
How often?	am pm	am pm	am pm	am pm	am pm	am pm	am pm
Brand/Dosage							
How often?	am pm	am pm	am pm	am pm	am pm	am pm	am pm
Brand/Dosage							
How often?	am pm	am pm	am pm	am pm	am pm	am pm	am pm
Brand/Dosage							
How often?	am pm	am pm	am pm	am pm	am pm	am pm	am pm
Brand/Dosage							
How often?	am pm	am pm	am pm	am pm	am pm	am pm	am pm

42

DAILY MEDICINE CONSUMPTION

Medicine	Date Sunday	Monday	Tuesday	Wednesday	Thursday	Friday	Saturday
Brand/Dosage	am / am	am / am	am / am	am / am	am / am	am / am	am / am
How often?	am / pm	am / pm	am / pm	am / pm	am / pm	am / pm	am / pm
Brand/Dosage	am / am	am / am	am / am	am / am	am / am	am / am	am / am
How often?	am / pm	am / pm	am / pm	am / pm	am / pm	am / pm	am / pm
Brand/Dosage	am / am	am / am	am / am	am / am	am / am	am / am	am / am
How often?	pm / pm	pm / pm	pm / pm	pm / pm	pm / pm	pm / pm	pm / pm
Brand/Dosage	am / am	am / am	am / am	am / am	am / am	am / am	am / am
How often?	pm / pm	pm / pm	pm / pm	pm / pm	pm / pm	pm / pm	pm / pm
Brand/Dosage	am / am	am / am	am / am	am / am	am / am	am / am	am / am
How often?	pm / pm	pm / pm	pm / pm	pm / pm	pm / pm	pm / pm	pm / pm

DAILY MEDICINE CONSUMPTION

Medicine	Sunday	Monday	Tuesday	Wednesday	Thursday	Friday	Saturday
Date							
Brand/Dosage							
How often?	am am / pm pm	am am / pm pm	am am / pm pm	am am / pm pm	am am / pm pm	am am / pm pm	am am / pm pm
Brand/Dosage							
How often?	am am / pm pm	am am / pm pm	am am / pm pm	am am / pm pm	am am / pm pm	am am / pm pm	am am / pm pm
Brand/Dosage							
How often?	am am / pm pm	am am / pm pm	am am / pm pm	am am / pm pm	am am / pm pm	am am / pm pm	am am / pm pm
Brand/Dosage							
How often?	am am / pm pm	am am / pm pm	am am / pm pm	am am / pm pm	am am / pm pm	am am / pm pm	am am / pm pm
Brand/Dosage							
How often?	am am / pm pm	am am / pm pm	am am / pm pm	am am / pm pm	am am / pm pm	am am / pm pm	am am / pm pm

Chapter 9

Next Appointment Form

When you take your Lifetime Medical Organizer to your doctor visits, the Next Appointment form allows you to record future doctor appointments. A calendar is another way to record appointments, and you may want to consider inserting one into your Lifetime Medical Organizer. Or, you can use the blank monthly calendar I have provided for your use. The Next Appointment form provides a quick comprehensive snapshot with all your doctor appointments on one page. With this quick reference, you can easily match medical insurance billing statements with appointment dates to ensure accuracy for medical services rendered.

My Experience

My mother keeps her doctors' appointments on a calendar hanging in the kitchen. She also writes birthdays and the dates of other social events on the calendar. This calendar helps manage her busy life, though it becomes less effective when trying to manage past, present, and future doctors' appointments.

For example, when I wanted to know the last time she visited her doctor, I had to go through all of the previous months of her calendar to find the sequence of appointments. Listing all of your appointments on one easy form summarizes the same information quickly.

How To

Show the appointment date, day, time, doctor name, and purpose on this form. Indicate whether the purpose is a regular or a follow-up appointment, a follow-up for a certain symptom, x-rays, outpatient surgery, laboratory and blood tests, or medical examinations. You might even record visits to your dentist. During an emergency situation, this form can help the attending doctor to know when you last saw a health care provider.

Questions to Consider

- How effective is my current method of recording doctor appointments?
- Could the person helping me easily determine when I last saw each of my doctors?

NEXT APPOINTMENT RECORD

Date	Day	Time	Name of Doctor	Reason for Visit
Date	Day	Time	Name of Doctor	Reason for Visit
Date	Day	Time	Name of Doctor	Reason for Visit
Date	Day	Time	Name of Doctor	Reason for Visit
Date	Day	Time	Name of Doctor	Reason for Visit
Date	Day	Time	Name of Doctor	Reason for Visit
Date	Day	Time	Name of Doctor	Reason for Visit
Date	Day	Time	Name of Doctor	Reason for Visit
Date	Day	Time	Name of Doctor	Reason for Visit

NEXT APPOINTMENT RECORD

Date	Day	Time	Name of Doctor	Reason for Visit
Date	Day	Time	Name of Doctor	Reason for Visit
Date	Day	Time	Name of Doctor	Reason for Visit
Date	Day	Time	Name of Doctor	Reason for Visit
Date	Day	Time	Name of Doctor	Reason for Visit
Date	Day	Time	Name of Doctor	Reason for Visit
Date	Day	Time	Name of Doctor	Reason for Visit
Date	Day	Time	Name of Doctor	Reason for Visit
Date	Day	Time	Name of Doctor	Reason for Visit

NEXT APPOINTMENT RECORD

Date	Day	Time	Name of Doctor	Reason for Visit
Date	Day	Time	Name of Doctor	Reason for Visit
Date	Day	Time	Name of Doctor	Reason for Visit
Date	Day	Time	Name of Doctor	Reason for Visit
Date	Day	Time	Name of Doctor	Reason for Visit
Date	Day	Time	Name of Doctor	Reason for Visit
Date	Day	Time	Name of Doctor	Reason for Visit
Date	Day	Time	Name of Doctor	Reason for Visit
Date	Day	Time	Name of Doctor	Reason for Visit

NEXT APPOINTMENT RECORD

Date	Day	Time	Name of Doctor	Reason for Visit
Date	Day	Time	Name of Doctor	Reason for Visit
Date	Day	Time	Name of Doctor	Reason for Visit
Date	Day	Time	Name of Doctor	Reason for Visit
Date	Day	Time	Name of Doctor	Reason for Visit
Date	Day	Time	Name of Doctor	Reason for Visit
Date	Day	Time	Name of Doctor	Reason for Visit
Date	Day	Time	Name of Doctor	Reason for Visit
Date	Day	Time	Name of Doctor	Reason for Visit

Month _____ Year _____

Monday	Tuesday	Wednesday	Thursday	Friday	Saturday	Sunday
☐	☐	☐	☐	☐	☐	☐
☐	☐	☐	☐	☐	☐	☐
☐	☐	☐	☐	☐	☐	☐
☐	☐	☐	☐	☐	☐	☐
☐	☐	☐	☐	☐	☐	☐

Month _____ Year _____

Monday	Tuesday	Wednesday	Thursday	Friday	Saturday	Sunday
☐	☐	☐	☐	☐	☐	☐
☐	☐	☐	☐	☐	☐	☐
☐	☐	☐	☐	☐	☐	☐
☐	☐	☐	☐	☐	☐	☐
☐	☐	☐	☐	☐	☐	☐

Chapter 10

Family Medical History Form

During a visit to a new doctor, an annual physical examination, or an application for life insurance, chances are you will be asked about your family medical history. Would you be able to recite this information from memory? Or are you like me and look toward the ceiling while trying to recall each family member's medical condition? Your doctor and insurance company need this information to decide whether you are "at risk" because of hereditary medical problems. Having this information easily available in your Lifetime Medical Organizer can help a doctor discover the root of your symptoms, especially if you are unable to communicate this history yourself.

My Experience

Although my parents lived in good health for most their lives, my grandparents, aunts, and uncles died from different illnesses. In addition, my brother lives with diabetes. As I grow older, my family medical history has become increasingly more important to me because I prefer to be proactive in my approach to staying healthy.

  I use the analogy of a car to remind myself of the importance of caring for my body. I can choose to wait for an indicator light to display before fixing my car, or I can schedule preventive maintenance to keep it running efficiently for longer periods. In the same way, I can take preventive measures to remain healthy for a longer period of time or wait until symptoms display before realizing that my body needs greater care. A major difference between my car and me is that I cannot trade in my body for a new one, and there is no indicator light that displays exactly what is wrong with my body.

How To

List the names of all family members that suffer some type of medical condition. If they are not living, show their age at death and what they died of or what other conditions they may have suffered. For example, they may have died of cancer and also suffered from high blood pressure. This information will bring awareness of potential hereditary risks to your health that you would normally not discuss with your doctor.

It is important to document whether the family member was a parent, grandparent, or great-grandparent because some medical conditions skip a generation. Your Family Medical History form should be something that you can discuss with all your family members to make sure it is as accurate as it can be.

Questions to Consider

*   Who is the best person to ask in my family about our family medical history?
*   Are there any patterns of illness in my family history that my doctor or emergency care provider should know about?

FAMILY MEDICAL HISTORY

FAMILY MEMBER	MEDICAL CONDITION
Name	Describe Condition
Relationship	
Age at Death	
Name	Describe Condition
Relationship	
Age at Death	
Name	Describe Condition
Relationship	
Age at Death	
Name	Describe Condition
Relationship	
Age at Death	
Name	Describe Condition
Relationship	
Age at Death	
Name	Describe Condition
Relationship	
Age at Death	
Name	Describe Condition
Relationship	
Age at Death	

FAMILY MEDICAL HISTORY

FAMILY MEMBER	MEDICAL CONDITION
Name Relationship Age at Death	Describe Condition
Name Relationship Age at Death	Describe Condition
Name Relationship Age at Death	Describe Condition
Name Relationship Age at Death	Describe Condition
Name Relationship Age at Death	Describe Condition
Name Relationship Age at Death	Describe Condition
Name Relationship Age at Death	Describe Condition

FAMILY MEDICAL HISTORY

FAMILY MEMBER	MEDICAL CONDITION
Name	Describe Condition
Relationship	
Age at Death	
Name	Describe Condition
Relationship	
Age at Death	
Name	Describe Condition
Relationship	
Age at Death	
Name	Describe Condition
Relationship	
Age at Death	
Name	Describe Condition
Relationship	
Age at Death	
Name	Describe Condition
Relationship	
Age at Death	
Name	Describe Condition
Relationship	
Age at Death	

FAMILY MEDICAL HISTORY

FAMILY MEMBER	MEDICAL CONDITION
Name Relationship Age at Death	Describe Condition
Name Relationship Age at Death	Describe Condition
Name Relationship Age at Death	Describe Condition
Name Relationship Age at Death	Describe Condition
Name Relationship Age at Death	Describe Condition
Name Relationship Age at Death	Describe Condition
Name Relationship Age at Death	Describe Condition

Chapter 11

Appointment Notes Form

The purpose of the Appointment Notes form is to summarize each of your doctor visits. It may not be necessary to write down entire conversations, but it is a good idea to highlight important notes for future reference. This point is emphasized when you are in the middle of an emergency or during a hospital stay that needs many visits to various doctors. This form can also be useful as a reference in case of any conflicts with medical bills.

My Experience

While my father was hospitalized, he had several doctors overseeing his care. Initially, my mother was the only one with him during the day, when most of the doctors came to check on him. After a while, it became difficult for my mother to remember everything each doctor said—especially when she had spoken with several doctors in a short period of time. When my sister and I were also present during a doctor visit, we recorded all the doctor's updates so my mother could discuss matters without having to worry about remembering every detail.

Another time, my mother asked a visiting friend to write down the notes while she spoke with the doctor. She found that it was a relief to have the information written instead of relying on memory. If no one was present with her during a visit, my mother would try her best to record notes on what the doctor was saying. Even if she did not capture everything in the conversation, her notes were usually enough for my sister and me to figure out what was said and follow up with the doctor if we had questions. Later in the evening, when my mother settled herself at home, she could review the notes and recap the day without distractions. In the same way, my sister and I could review updates and share the same information with extended family and friends. Also, we could reference these notes whenever we discussed future updates with doctors.

How To

Establish a chronological history of doctor meetings by completing a form for each visit. It is up to you to decide how comprehensive you want the notes to be on the form. For less frequent visits, you may want to consider writing a quick summary. Or you may feel that more information is necessary, depending on the outcome of your visit. Whatever approach you decide, it is important for you to *write legibly* so others can understand and read your handwriting.

When visiting your doctor's office, ask the doctor or the nurse to provide help in documenting the most important information from the visit. By discussing your Lifetime Medical Organizer, information or concerns can be brought up and answered for documentation. With their assistance, you can develop a good method for recording this information on the form.

Often we hesitate admitting to doctors that we do not understand some of their recommendations and advice. Perhaps we don't want to "look dumb." Most doctors are willing to translate their complex terminology so we can understand it, but often this concern is not addressed until we ask for clarification. By communicating better with our doctors, we will have greater peace of mind and a better understanding about our health.

Questions to Consider

- How can I use my meeting notes to be more proactive during my next doctor visit?
- Do I understand everything my doctors have told me? (If not, ask for clarification.)

APPOINTMENT NOTES

APPOINTMENT	DOCTOR
Date	Name
Reason	Specialty

APPOINTMENT SUMMARY

APPOINTMENT NOTES

APPOINTMENT	DOCTOR
Date	Name
Reason	Specialty

APPOINTMENT SUMMARY

APPOINTMENT NOTES

APPOINTMENT	DOCTOR
Date	Name
Reason	Specialty

APPOINTMENT SUMMARY

APPOINTMENT NOTES

APPOINTMENT	DOCTOR
Date	Name
Reason	Specialty

APPOINTMENT SUMMARY

Chapter 12

Journal Notes Form

A journal lets one freely express thoughts, reflections, and questions on paper. People journal their eating habits, exercise routines, prayers, personal improvement, and events of the day. In the same way, the Journal Notes form in your Lifetime Medical Organizer allows you to record changes resulting from the medicine you are taking or changes in your physical or emotional condition. You can also use this form to write down questions you want to ask your doctor on the next visit.

My Experience

I asked my mother to list changes in my father's eating habits, bowel movements, temperature, and any other information she thought was important for review when the hospice nurse visited. Even when my mother had a question that was not urgent, she wrote it on this form. Sometimes when the hospice nurse made follow-up visits or telephone calls, my sister and I could immediately provide updates and information by referencing the Lifetime Medical Organizer. We didn't have to bother my mother to get this information because it was all in the organizer for easy reference. If there was any information from the dialogue with the nurse, we immediately recorded it on the appointment notes or made comments on the journal notes.

How To

List any changes or observations and the date of occurrence on the form. Also, record any questions you may want to ask of health care providers, family members, and others. If you see something inconsistent or have a concern, write it down no matter how minor it may seem at the time. Many symptoms show up prior to a condition and become progressively worse. By recording the occurrence of these symptoms in the journal, a trained doctor might foresee a condition and be able to address it before it becomes a major problem.

Questions to Consider

- Do I have any concerns or questions to note for future discussions with my doctors?
- Have I noticed any inconsistencies or changes in my health or eating habits recently?

JOURNAL NOTES

Indicate any changes to medication, behavior, physical changes, questions to ask the doctor, etc.

List observations or questions to ask	Date

List observations or questions to ask	Date

List observations or questions to ask	Date

List observations or questions to ask	Date

List observations or questions to ask	Date

List observations or questions to ask	Date

List observations or questions to ask	Date

JOURNAL NOTES

Indicate any changes to medication, behavior, physical changes, questions to ask the doctor, etc.

List observations or questions to ask	Date

List observations or questions to ask	Date

List observations or questions to ask	Date

List observations or questions to ask	Date

List observations or questions to ask	Date

List observations or questions to ask	Date

List observations or questions to ask	Date

JOURNAL NOTES

Indicate any changes to medication, behavior, physical changes, questions to ask the doctor, etc.

List observations or questions to ask	Date

List observations or questions to ask	Date

List observations or questions to ask	Date

List observations or questions to ask	Date

List observations or questions to ask	Date

List observations or questions to ask	Date

List observations or questions to ask	Date

JOURNAL NOTES

Indicate any changes to medication, behavior, physical changes, questions to ask the doctor, etc.

List observations or questions to ask	Date

List observations or questions to ask	Date

List observations or questions to ask	Date

List observations or questions to ask	Date

List observations or questions to ask	Date

List observations or questions to ask	Date

List observations or questions to ask	Date

Chapter 13

Wills and Trusts

Wills and trusts are legal documents that help decide how to manage personal assets according to your wishes. There are *living wills* that provide directions if you should become incapacitated and *final wills* that are executed after your death. Most legal documents should be safely secured in storage devices such as a safety deposit box or lockable file cabinet. It is recommended that a copy of these documents be included in your Lifetime Medical Organizer for quick reference.

If your legal documents are stored in a device that needs a key, a password, or a combination that only you know, the person providing help for you will have a difficult time getting these documents and managing your affairs. In addition, most people forget about their legal documents once they are safely stored away. By keeping copies of these documents in your Lifetime Medical Organizer, you can easily reference them periodically to determine if your initial bequests are still your intentions today. You can indicate the location of the key, password, or combination to the storage device in your organizer as well.

If you are not familiar with a will or trust, my friend Bart Koza, an estate planning attorney and certified public accountant, provides the legal expertise to guide you in the chapters that discuss legal documents. He explains estate planning as the process of deciding who will inherit your assets when you pass away. No matter who we are, we all own some assets. Regardless of how many assets you have, you cannot take them with you. Each state has its own specific laws deciding how assets will be divided when people pass away if there are no terms in a will. To ensure that your assets are passed along to those you want to receive them, a will or trust is extremely important.

A Will

Most people are familiar with a last will and testament, commonly known as simply a "will." A will is a document that indicates how you want to divide your assets at the time of your death. In addition, a will can name a guardian or conservator if your surviving child/children are under the age of 18 years old and the other parent (or legal guardian) is also deceased. Once a will is set up, it does not become active until you die. A will has limitations that may not make it the most fitting legal document for your situation.

A Trust

In comparison, a trust works similar to a will in that it identifies how to divide your assets at the time of your death. There are other benefits that only a trust can provide. A trust can reduce estate taxes and probate, where a will cannot. Most states will view a trust as an entity or a company. Therefore, when you pass away, the trust becomes a separate entity that represents your estate on your behalf. The biggest *misconception* people have about a trust is that once they sign the trust, all the assets are automatically linked to it. This is not the case.

When setting up a will or trust, you should consider consulting an estate planning attorney for comprehensive guidance in the setup and management. If you do not have a will or trust, consider taking advantage of a free consultation with a professional to get more information. If you wait until an emergency arises, you may not be competent or able to begin these documents. If that is the case, you could lose control of how your assets will be divided or perhaps even who will care for your children.

My Experience

As a financial professional, I have come across situations with families where the laws governing wills and trusts have helped some and hurt some, depending on the situation. For example, you may want a specific piece of jewelry bequeathed to your favorite niece or granddaughter, but your will or trust does not show the same intent. Therefore, this piece of jewelry may be divided differently if you have not provided for your bequests.

Another example involves parents who procrastinate to create legal documents to show who will care for young children upon the death of one or both parents. If both parents were to die simultaneously, the person named as guardian for the children may not be the one the parents would have preferred.

If you own any assets, or have children, you should seek the advice of an estate planning attorney about the best way to protect your most valuable possessions. In matters of emergencies, these documents can make the process of managing or settling your estate convenient for your loved ones.

Questions to Consider

- Do I have a will or trust?
- Have I stipulated how my assets will be divided or who cares for my children if I am incapacitated or suffer a premature death?
- (If you already have a will or trust) How long has it been since I reviewed it with my attorney?

Chapter 14

Durable General Power of Attorney Form

If you are unable to make sound judgments or decisions because of illness, someone will need to help you with your personal affairs. The Lifetime Medical Organizer should be the first place someone looks for a copy of your Durable General Power of Attorney form. The power of attorney is a legal document indicating who you want to oversee every aspect of your life and possessions during incapacity or incompetency. Having a copy of your power of attorney in your Lifetime Medical Organizer will speed up any matters without delay. During an emergency, decisions can be made more quickly if this document is available at a moment's notice.

If you do not have a power of attorney in place when you need it most, your situation may require the intervention of the courts. Anytime your loved ones have to go to court on your behalf, it will involve much time and could become costly for them. A power of attorney is an important document to create—it is also a powerful document. Therefore, be careful about who you name because the person you designate will be allowed to have immediate access to all of your personal belongings and financial accounts unless your power of attorney states otherwise.

My Experience

My parents set up legal documents many years before my father's illness, so there was no interruption in accessing or managing financial affairs when he became incapacitated. I recently learned of a woman who was diagnosed with Alzheimer's disease, and her power of attorney named her eldest son, who lived in another state far away, to manage her affairs. The power of attorney had been created many years ago and had never been updated. However, at the time of her illness, this woman's younger son lived with her and took care of her affairs. On learning that his older brother was the power of attorney, resentment set in. Since there were lingering conflicts between the sons, it was difficult for each to manage and communicate in the best interest of their mother, and the physical distance added another level of challenge to the situation.

You should consider reviewing your power of attorney documents to decide if there are any conflicts between the person you appointed as your attorney-in-fact and other members of your family. Also, some children may express no interest in accepting the role, while others may need to be made aware. In addition, it is important to review the power of attorney from time to time to make sure the appointed person is still alive or is consistent with your current wishes.

Questions to Consider

- Who is the person most interested in managing my affairs if I cannot decide for myself?
- If I already created a power of attorney document, does it need to be reviewed or updated?
- Should I discuss my power of attorney document with my family?

Chapter 15

Advanced Health Care Directives

The Advanced Health Care Directive form is similar to a Durable General Power of Attorney form, but covers only medical issues. The medical directive is a document that allows you to appoint someone to aid in your medical decisions if you are unable to decide for yourself. In addition, the medical directive allows you to decide in advance if you want to remain on a life support machine if you become permanently disabled. You can also make personal choices on other medical issues, such as pain relief, organ donation, and burial instructions.

The day may come when the people who love you must decide whether or not to turn off your life support. Your health care directive is your opportunity to lessen their guilt or concern. The directive will provide your loved ones with peace of mind that their choices will be the best decisions for you.

By now, you should have the understanding that copies of your documents are important to keep in your Lifetime Medical Organizer. If you have not established these documents yet, consider consulting an estate planning attorney as soon as possible.

My Experience

I have accompanied clients and their attorneys in meetings where one spouse immediately decides what he or she wants to do in a situation that calls for a health care directive, while the other spouse is distraught at the thought of having to make such an important decision in advance. There are many reasons people choose to stop life support, but there are no right or wrong decisions, only the decision you make for yourself and feel is right for you.

You may want to consider explaining your wishes to your family. This will eliminate or lessen any guilt or burden when it becomes necessary to carry out the health care directive. These subjects are never easy to discuss, but open communication will help to ensure that your choices are carried out even if it requires a difficult decision.

Questions to Consider

- Am I doing this for me or to lessen the burden for my loved ones?
- How can I best explain my intentions so my family will respect my choices?

Chapter 16

Other Important Documents

At this point, you have a pretty good idea of how to develop the life and health sections of your Lifetime Medical Organizer. The forms, directions, and descriptions provided in this book are the essentials to help you get started. Now you are ready to include additional information that is specific to your situation. Some of the tips I share below are easy for you to build upon in your organizer at your discretion. Customizing your organizer gives it a personal touch that defines your personality. Visit our website at www.lifemedorganizer.com for more information and ideas and to download forms that will help you to preserve your organizer for a lifetime.

Medical Release Form

A Medical Release form is provided to keep handy in your organizer. Should medical professionals require additional records from you, this form quickly allows them to gather this information from third party sources. Please note that some providers may have their own similar form for you to complete.

Personal Profile

In the event you misplace your organizer during a doctor or hospital visit, this page will quickly help the finder to identify and contact you promptly.

Business Card Holder

Consider adding a plastic business card sheet to store the important business contacts that correspond to the contacts listed in your organizer.

Photo I.D.

It is a good idea to insert a picture of yourself to add a personal touch to your organizer.

Divider Tabs

Divider tabs are helpful to separate each form for quicker access and easier identification.

Caretaker Notification

Complete the Caretaker Notification form and keep it with your Lifetime Medical Organizer so the caretaker will have all the information needed during an emergency.

Travel Itinerary

If you travel, it is a good idea to include the Travel Itinerary form in your Lifetime Medical Organizer. Whether the organizer is traveling with you or is safe at home, a set of itinerary information becomes a quick and handy reference for family members or friends, especially if you are single.

Health Coverage Information

Insert copies of your medical, dental, vision, and prescription drug cards and other medical condition cards in your Lifetime Medical Organizer. If you become unconscious or unable to speak, this information can assist in medical attention.

Other Medical Conditions Report

If you are monitoring other types of medical conditions and are keeping a record of your progress and diagnosis, make sure you include this information in your Lifetime Medical Organizer. Building an organizer with information relative to all medical conditions establishes a comprehensive and proactive approach to organizing your life and health needs.

Insurance Claims and Forms

Keep a copy of all insurance claims and required forms from the hospital in your Lifetime Medical Organizer for easier reference and reconciliation of billing invoices.

RELEASE OF CERTAIN HEALTH-RELATED INFORMATION

By signing below, I am authorizing _____ to release, or make available, certain information regarding my health or medical records. I understand that information regarding sensitive medical histories will not be released or made available unless I have initialed below. This includes, but is not limited to, HIV, alcohol or drug abuse, mental and psychiatric disorders, cognitive impairments, or medical information that may be restricted by law.

In addition, I understand that I may send a written notice to revoke this authorization at any time. I further understand that any action already taken in advance of this revocation cannot be reversed.

PROVIDE INFORMATION TO:

_____

_____

_____

Information to be included (please initial):

_____ Entire medical records (information about my past, present, or future physical or mental health or condition; and any related diagnosis, treatment, or prognosis related to the same.

_____ Medical history from (date) _____ to (date) _____

_____ HIV

_____ Alcohol or drug abuse

_____ Mental and psychiatric disorders

_____ Cognitive impairments

This authorization shall expire on _____ or one year after the date indicated below.

_____   _____
Date   Print Name

_____   _____
Date of Birth   Signature

(Insert picture here)

This Lifetime Medical Organizer belongs to:

Name _____

Address _____

_____

City, State, Zip _____

Home Phone No. _____

Cell Phone No. _____

Fax No. _____

E-mail Address _____

Medical Provider _____

Group # _____

Vision # _____

Prescription Drug # _____

Dental Provider _____

Group #_____

Blood Type _____

CARETAKER NOTIFICATION

I (We) will be at the following location:

Name   Date

Location

Address

Phone No.

Time   From   am/pm   To   am/pm

Name   Date

Location

Address

Phone No.

Time   From   am/pm   To   am/pm

Instructions:

CARETAKER NOTIFICATION

I (We) will be at the following location:

Name   Date

Location

Address

Phone No.

Time   From   am/pm   To   am/pm

Name   Date

Location

Address

Phone No.

Time   From   am/pm   To   am/pm

Instructions:

CARETAKER NOTIFICATION

I (We) will be at the following location:

Name   Date

Location

Address

Phone No.

Time   From   am/pm   To   am/pm

Name   Date

Location

Address

Phone No.

Time   From   am/pm   To   am/pm

Instructions:

CARETAKER NOTIFICATION

I (We) will be at the following location:

Name   Date

Location

Address

Phone No.

Time   From   am/pm   To   am/pm

Name   Date

Location

Address

Phone No.

Time   From   am/pm   To   am/pm

Instructions:

NOTES

_____

_____

_____

_____

_____

_____

_____

_____

_____

_____

_____

_____

_____

_____

_____

_____

_____

_____

_____

_____

_____

_____

_____

_____

_____

_____

_____

_____

NOTES

_____

_____

_____

_____

_____

_____

_____

_____

_____

_____

_____

_____

_____

_____

_____

_____

_____

_____

_____

_____

_____

_____

_____

_____

_____

_____

_____

_____

_____

NOTES

NOTES

Download forms and other helpful information at

www.lifemedorganizer.com

About the Author

Sandra J. Yorong

Sandra Yorong is a financial advisor and a former trust officer and investment portfolio manager with 15 years of experience in the financial industry. Sandra is a volunteer guild member with a nonprofit organization for many years, gives her time helping others, and is actively involved with her church. She brings her personal story, her experience with helping clients, and her involvement with helping people in need to reach out to the reader in a realistic and relatable approach.

Known for her ability to develop systems to organize just about anything, Sandra hopes this book will give people the resources to make things easier to manage with important matters of life and health. In this way, Sandra hopes to achieve her personal goal of helping and inspring others in some small way .

Sandra can be reached at www.lifemedorganizer.com.

About the Co-Author

Richard Schuttler, Ph.D.

Richard Schuttler is an international public speaker, educator, and author. He has 20 years of diversified, domestic, and international management/leadership improvement expertise within academic, federal/state governments, and Fortune 1000 environments developing strategies and implementation methods. He has mentored executives, faculty, and students from around the world in various professional settings.

Richard is the author of *Laws of Communication*. He is the co-author of *Million Dollar Attitude* and *Working in Groups: Communication Principles and Strategies* and a contributing author in *Online Assessment and Measurement: Foundations and Challenge*.

Richard owns Organizational Troubleshooter, LLC from offices in Honolulu, Hawaii, and Phoenix, Arizona. He can be reached at www.orgtroubleshooter.org.

Edwards Brothers Malloy
Oxnard, CA USA
February 5, 2015